TABLE OF CONTENTS

INTRODUCTION

CHAPTER 1 : HOW TO ACTIVATE WOMEN VAGINAL PLEASURE?

CHAPTER 2; DO YOU KNOW THAT YOGURT CAN INCREASE SEXUAL PERFORMANCE?

CHAPTER 3: WOMEN: WHAT ARE THE PREFERRED METHODS FOR INTENSE PLEASURE?

CHAPTER 4 :THE 3 TIPS TO HAVE A LIFETIME GREAT SEX

CHAPTER 5: SOME TIPS ON HOW TO USE THE PREGNANCY CONTRACEPTIVE PIL

CHAPTER 6: HOW TO HAVE A GREAT SLEEP WITH SEX?

CHAPTER 7 : BEWARE ORAL SEX LOVERS !!!

CHAPTER 8 ; HOW TO MAINTAIN YOUR BRAIN?

CHAPTER 8 : HOW YOUR COFFEE CAN MAKE YOUR BELLY BIG

CHAPTER 10: 5 FOODS THAT PUMP OUR ENERGY

CHAPTER 11 : TIPS TO EDUCATE YOUR CHILD TO FOLLOW THE RULES.

CHAPTER 12: BE CAREFUL: CARBONATED WATER CAN MAKE YOU HUNGRY.

CHAPTER 13: WHAT IS PRECONCEPTION CONSULTATION AND WHY IS IT SO IMPORTANT STEP?

CHAPTER 14: DO NOT GIVE CODEINE OR TRAMADOL TO A CHILD

CHAPTER 15: HOW TO CHANGE THE AGE OF YOUR HEART

CHAPTER 16: WHAT ARE THE VITAMINS AND MINERALS FOR CHILDREN BETWEEN 1 TO 3 YEARS OLD?

INTRODUCTION

In this book I share some of my successful articles on my blog www.jpsante.com.
This short book aim is to make your sexual life better. So I strongly advise you not to only read the chapter but apply the advices & tips gained. let's go .

CHAPTER ONE

HOW TO ACTIVATE WOMEN VAGINAL PLEASURE?

Here, I will talk about the female pleasure, and I think it will interest many men who often have difficulty understanding how women function. And too, I would say that women sometimes have trouble understanding how they function themselves.

So how begins the awakening of the vagina, and how is it different from the penis one?
JPsante: The vagina is a hidden place and closed in part by the hymen. So it has no contact with the outside before the first sexual relationship. The vagina of a little girl did not enjoy any sensory experience when first time. It is a virgin.
The penis of a boy, on the contrary, experiencing lots of adventures. Before birth, it is already in contact with the amniotic fluid in the womb. After birth, it is in contact with the bath water, the hand of the person who washes, change her diapers, in contact with his clothes, and of course, the touch of his hand, or to urinate, or just for fun, since it is close at hand!

These sexual areas do not have the same history in men and in women. What will be the difference in sexual life?
JPsante: It's simple at first intercourse, a young man knows his penis. And his penis went through experiences. For the first time, the girl does not know her vagina. And she will not feel anything. So, the first time the boy will easily have a pleasure and orgasm during penetration and movements back and forth. The girl is often disappointed. She may feel pain during the rupture of the hymen, but not necessarily, and then she often says, "but I do not feel anything! Yet this is what we talk so much! »
And she thinks as she is abnormal. "I should have fun," she thinks ... In reality, 95% of women do not have an orgasm the first time, although there are some lucky!

The first time, she does not feel much, but then what?
JPsante: Then there are several possibilities. Either she thinks she is not normal and often it simulates pleasure. She thinks her partner will be offended or will think she has a problem if she does not show fun. It's annoying because it's not going to be in a real intimacy with each other and move towards pleasure.
Either she said, "Well, I did not feel much this first time, but still, it sounds interesting. This was only the first time, I'll see how it goes next time ... "And in this case, she agreed to from almost nothing. And she's right. Her vagina has no experience, but willing to learn! The vagina has everything to give her the pleasure. It just needs to learn and get experiences.

How does the vagina learn to have the pleasure?

JPsante: It happens in several ways.
• First of all the senses. The woman had better watch what she feels in her vagina. Is it the heat? Pressure? Friction? A tickling? A kind of thrill, itching? And where? On the front, the back, at the bottom, near the entrance? It is from the sensations she observed inside it will get to know and integrate these sensations which encourages them to turn into pleasure. It is as if we had the pleasure cable between sex and brain. So now, to self-observe and enjoy the sensations of pleasure, even minimal.
• Then there is the sexual practice. The variety of movements back and forth is important. That is if the partner is doing its best to help awaken her vagina to pleasure. It could for example - very slow movements sometimes, sometimes fast movements. - Sometimes very superficial movements barely penetrating the vagina, sometimes deep movements - movements that sometimes abut on one side of the vagina to pressure, sometimes gliding movements in the axis of the vagina.
• And then caresses the vagina with fingers eventually. With all these variations, the vagina will eroticize as they say. It will learn to enjoy the fun.

How long does it take for a woman who started her sex life, to get vaginal pleasure?
JPsante: It is very variable and very unfair. For some women, some sex intercourses, pleasure is already present. For others, it will take weeks, months or years. But be aware that even if the fun comes soon enough, there is always more fun to explore! And long term, we know that only about 35% of women have vaginal orgasms, even if others are also feeling pleasure.

And when the pleasure is taking time, there are women who have very little sexual pleasure?
JPsante: Not necessarily, because we are only talking about the vagina. We have the female clitoris, labia minora and the entire vulva that can also be sources of pleasure! We'll talk about another time!

CHAPTER TWO

DO YOU KNOW THAT YOGURT CAN INCREASE SEXUAL PERFORMANCE?

The world has still its hidden secrets. MIT researchers wanted to study the relationship between yogurt consumption and obesity. Surprisingly, they have discovered that these products can have unexpected effects on sexuality! Good or bad news? Let us find out in coming lines

Members of the Massachusetts Institute of Technology (MIT), the scientists analyzed the behaviors of 40 female mice and 40 male mice. Some have received high-fat foods, others have adapted food for them and a third group, vanilla yogurt. And there, surprise! Males in the latter group were visibly much more sexually stimulated than other rodents. They were faster to inseminate females. They also took a step that showed their testicles, which were larger than those of other male mice! Finally, their hairs were more silky and thicker

According to Susan Erdman, oncologist biologist, the benefit of yogurt on libido may be related to its content of probiotics . New research will be conducted to study the effect on humans.

CHAPTER THREE

WOMEN: WHAT ARE THE PREFERRED METHODS FOR INTENSE PLEASURE?

Some women are cheating on their partners for the simple motif of not been satisfied during the sexual act. This suggested that sexual act may require some know-hows from men to be on the top of their job.
Why not ask the women what are their preferred methods that will bring heaven down.

Many people believe that the women are very satisfied when the sexual act lasts long. But, it seems, it is not true as we think. A new study published in the medical journal Sex & Marital Therapy explains that contrary to what many men think, it is not the penetration time that counts to make a woman's pleasure stronger. Indeed in this survey, 82% of the women confirmed that vaginal penetration is not enough for them to reach the orgasm.

You will be asking what do women really need?
To come out with this revelation, American researchers interviewed 1055 women between the ages of 18 and 94. The study revealed that 36% said they needed clitoral stimulation to reach seventh heaven. Added to this, it is a must to add a time necessary to raise the excitement, the emotional load, and to feel loved by its partner.

Debby Herbenick, director of the Sexuality Research Section at Indiana University (USA) and author of the study points out that if men are to learn what women really want, it will be the duty of women to show them. Women need caresses, yes, but even if this loses spontaneity, do not hesitate to show your partner the right way to do it or to make him understand when he reaches the goal.

CHAPTER FOUR

THE 3 TIPS TO HAVE A LIFETIME GREAT SEX

Yes, we are in 2018. To start the year on a good note, I decided to talk about the sexual act. The act that helps us to maintain our mental stability. Being stable in mind, you can achieve great things. So how to really enjoy sexual act? Simply check out the three tips of sex therapist Tracey Cox to have fun in bed ... every time!

Preliminaries, positions, outfits, places ... If making love is already part of a common desire of two people who attract each other, there are some little basics to know to optimize these rascals reunion and especially have fun. On the English *Dailymail* website, sex therapist Tracey Cox advises three things:

• Make love at least twice a week: According to this specialist, it is important to spend time with the couple to get together. The idea is not to make it a marathon sex, but to caress regularly. Without forgetting that the more we make love, the more we want it.

• Do not hesitate to say "no": "Stop listening to what is said everywhere: the desire of everyone goes up and down" insists the sex therapist Tracey Cox. And it's better to refuse to make love than to force yourself and create discomfort with your partner. Moreover, on this point, the expert advises saying rather "Let's wait for this weekend to find us without rushing" rather than "I really have something else to think". In addition, refusing can create some sexual excitement with your partner and spice up your intimate life. Play it!

• Stay faithful: "No one can deny that the libido is relaunched by a new partner, even more so when the relationship is taking place. But once you are used to the new body of the other, the" new "side fades "recalls Trace Cox. So unless you want to multiply unofficial partners all your life, more work to improve your sexual relations with the same person. "Being unfaithful to keep a dynamic sex life rarely works, and it's exhausting," the specialist concludes.

If you are going through a sexually complicated time with your partner, know that there are a few things that can rekindle the flame and desire between you. Dr. Gérard Leleu, sexologist, explained recently that it was good for the couple to make love in different places, to create the show with candles or music, to remain attractive even on weekends, not to forget the kisses and caresses outside the sex act and to privilege the quality to the sex act more than the quantity.

CHAPTER FIVE

SOME TIPS ON HOW TO USE THE PREGNANCY CONTRACEPTIVE PILL

I heard saying, I took my contraceptive pill but I got pregnant. Why so? Today JPsante will give some tips on using the pill.
Birth control pills are one of the most used contraceptives. And the question is how to use it? There are several kinds of pills and I'm going to talk today about the classic low-dose pills frequently used.
Those in the form of pads 21 tablets, with a 7-day break between each wafer.

FIRST OF ALL, HOW TO USE IT WHEN WE WANT TO TAKE THE PILL?
JPsante: You should see a doctor that will make a prescription. It is he who decides whether or not a woman can take the pill medically, and it is he who decides which pill to prescribe. This is never a woman who says "I want this or that pill" ...

WHY IS THE DOCTOR WHO DECIDES EVERYTHING?
JPsante: Simply for the woman health. It should not take the pill if it has against indications or takes a pill that would not be appropriate. But it is not provided the doctor decides everything. He must decide in agreement with the woman. If for instance, it has against indications for the pill, he suggests other means of contraception and chose together the appropriate one.

ONCE ONE HAS ITS ORDER PILL, WHAT DO WE DO?
JPsante: We will buy it in pharmacies. Then there are 2 ways to begin. We can expect the first day of her period. And in this case, we will be protected against an unwanted pregnancy from taking the first tablet.
Either we want to start faster immediately, regardless of the day. In this case, we will be protected from unwanted pregnancy had until 8th-day pill. The first 7 days are at risk and must therefore either avoid sex or use condoms.

AND WHEN WE STOP THE PILL FOR 7 DAYS OFF. IS IT A RISK PERIOD OF PREGNANCY?
JPsante: The pill also protects during the 7 days off, as long as you take the next pack. If you end a pill plate and do not take into account the next pack, consider that it is no longer protected after stopping the last tablet.

AND WHEN WE FORGET THE PILL, WHAT SHOULD WE DO? HOW TO REACT?
JPsante: Before saying what to do, I will explain how the pill works for a great understanding. In fact, take the pill for 7 consecutive days to block the ovulation. Similarly, we must stop the pill more than 7 days for the ovulation to be triggered.

- So, if we forget the pill in the first week, it is very high risk. Because we just made 7 days stop plus forgot days. Forgetting is worse than the first day of the process. It causes a relatively high risk of pregnancy. And during the first week, there is also a risk. So if an omission occurs during the first week of the process, it is necessary to quickly take the next day pill and more if we had sex during the previous 5 days. And consider that we will be protected again after 7-day pill taken without forgetting. Therefore, for 7 days, avoid sex or use a condom.

- If you forget the pill in the middle of the process, it does not matter. Indeed, it makes you forget one day, maybe two or three, but rarely 7. So ovulation continues to be blocked. There is nothing special to do.

- If you forget the pill during the last week, is at risk, because it will stop the pill for 7 days. This will make 7 days without pills (the stopping days) + forgot days, so a risk of triggering ovulation. So to avoid taking a risk, it must bind the next pack without stopping. So, instead of a stop of 7 days, we will have one stop corresponding to oblivion. If one connects the next pack without stopping, there will be no risk of pregnancy.

BUT ALL THE OMISSIONS ARE NOT SERIOUS. AN OVERSIGHT UNDER 12 HOURS IS OF NO CONSEQUENCE ...
JPsante: It's true. One should also not forget to mention but offset. It may well shift the pill within 12 hours, it continues to be effective. So if you forget to take it and that one finds out 4 hours later, simply take it and there's no problem.

AND WHEN YOU SMOKE, IS TO AVOID THE PILL?
JPsante: It's better not to smoke if you take the pill because strokes are increased when smoking is associated with the pill. However, for a very young woman, these accidents are rare. We consider that after 35 years, a doctor should not prescribe the pill to a woman who smokes. Before this age, if it is desired to run the risk, she has the right to be informed provided.

AND WHEN A WOMAN DOES NOT HAVE MENSTRUATION ON THE PILL, IS IT POSSIBLE?
JPsante: If a woman does not want to bleed between two packs, she can continue them without stopping. Beware that bleedings under the pill are not actually menstruations. It is withdrawal bleeding associated with stopping the hormones in the pill.

AND WHEN YOU WANT TO STOP THE PILL, HOW TO DO?
JPsante: It's very simple, do not take the next pack. And if we stop being in the process, it is also possible. Knowing that from the stop, we will no longer be protected against an unwanted pregnancy.

CHAPTER SIX

HOW TO HAVE A GREAT SLEEP WITH SEX?

Australian researchers say that having sex before sleep is the solution to a peaceful sleep.

Not easy to disconnect screens before sleeping! Researchers at the Adelaide Australian Sleep Clinic have found that having sex before bedtime is the key to a good night's sleep

An Orgasm To Sleep Well
The authors conducted a survey of 460 participants aged 18 to 70 years. One of the authors of the study, Michele Lastella, told the English media *Dailymail* that sex has the power to improve the quality of sleep. For proof, 64% of those surveyed in their study said they had better sleep after having sex with an orgasm. Moreover, seeing the satisfaction of the other partner would provide the personal satisfaction that would help to sleep peacefully.

Keep The Phone Away, Far Away From The Bed!
Conversely, one thing is to ban before falling asleep: the use of phone screens, computer or tablet. "It is increasingly difficult for adults to disconnect before falling asleep," confirms Michele Lastelle. But "there is strong evidence suggesting replacing screen time with time spent on sex." Nobody doubts it! Especially since an American study of 30 men, 20 of whom had already had erectile dysfunction in the last six months and 10 never, showed that those who had erection problems kept their phone with them on average 4 hours a day against just under 2 hours for others. "This pilot study shows that there may be a relationship between cell phone use and erectile dysfunction," said Badereddin Mohamad Al-Ali, the lead author of the research, which also shows that total exposure time on the phone is much more important than the short duration of intense exposure during the phone call. " Go, gentlemen, pick up a little!

CHAPTER SEVEN

BEWARE ORAL SEX LOVERS !!!

Men who have practiced oral sex on more than 5 women have a risk of ENT cancers. Research outcomes explain that the risk of ENT cancers increases significantly in people who have practiced on more than 5 partners.

Before delving into the matter, what is ENT cancers?
According to Wikipedia, ENT cancers is a group of cancers that start within the mouth, nose, throat, larynx, sinuses or salivary glands. Symptoms may include a lump or sore that does not heal, a sore throat that does not go away, trouble swallowing, or a change in the voice.

According to the Arc Foundation for Cancer Research, 14,706 new cases of digestive tract cancers were diagnosed in 2015. A new study done by American researchers at the John Hopkins Bloomberg School of Public Health (USA) found that men who gave cunnilingus to more than 5 partners during their lifetime are more likely to get this type of cancer too called ENT cancers. Practicing it on more than 5 partners, oral sex lovers have 15% risk of getting ENT cancers

How did they reach this outcome?
JPsante: To reach this conclusion, the researchers analyzed data from 13,089 volunteers between the ages of 20 and 69 who participated in a Papillomavirus (HPV) screening program. The results show for men the risk is increased by 4% among non-smokers who have already given oral sex to 4 different partners. Beyond the percentage reaches 7.1%. The biggest risk is for smokers who have had more than 5 partners because it increases significantly to 15%.
On the other hand, for women, regardless of their number of partners, they have a rather low risk of contracting HPV.

CHAPTER NINE

HOW TO MAINTAIN YOUR BRAIN?

I have regularly heard these phrases in my close circle...I have it on the tip of the tongue it will come back to me ... For 2 days I'm looking for the title of this movie ... I am still looking for my keys. What am I coming to do in this places

Memory "holes" can be mere signs of fatigue, overwork or stress, and everyone has it! However, do not forget the regular memory loss or do not underestimate what your entourage is saying about your ability to memorize. Over the years, our brain can become less efficient. It is then more difficult to learn, memorize and use new information. But the cognitive decline is not necessarily an obligatory passage provided you take care of your brain, coach it, just as you have to do with your whole body.

BY THE WAY ... WHAT IS MEMORY?
Memory is the ability to learn something, to memorize it and it is also the ability to remember it (restitution)!
• Short-term memory, or working memory, allows us to remember
for a few seconds, for example, a date or a phone number. We solicit it at every moment.
• Long-term memory accumulates memories over the years.

DOES THE BRAIN HAVE A SEX?
The answer is yes. The brain of the man is indeed different from that of the woman. More exactly, an American study1 has shown that we do not function in exactly the same way because we are connected in a different way. (Well, we knew it!)
Men would be better at perceiving and coordinating actions, while women seem to have more social skills, to be able to memorize. They are also multitasking. I reassure everyone ... The researchers specify that we should not generalize these results because each being can have in him both male and female. And voila!

NOW HOW TO MAINTAIN YOUR BRAIN?

Coach your memory
All intellectual activities contribute to the preservation of memory, provided that they are practiced without stress and with pleasure. Among them, reading is a particularly complete exercise to stimulate one's memory.

Design your exercises!

Exercise 1: Do you think you cannot remember a funny story you are told? Take a notebook and write down each new story. When you have a moment re-read what you have written. So you can tell it your turn!

Exercise 2: To develop your immediate memory and help your brain to quickly retain new information, observe for a few seconds a list of words, such as a shopping list or tasks to perform, try to remember them and then recite them in order.

Zen, let's stay zen ...
Relaxation or yoga sessions can help you better manage stress.
Yoga is an asset for the efficiency of your brain

Yoga combines physical postures, breathing techniques, meditation or relaxation. It touches both the mind and the physical. His practice seems to have a beneficial effect on cognitive functions.

Run, swim, and ride bicycle regularly
Playing sports helps oxygenate the brain and provide all the nutrients it needs, improving cognitive function.
Walking, swimming, riding or running regularly, it's up to you!

Do not stay alone!
Loneliness would have a negative impact on memory. On the other hand, go out, see one's friends, invest in an associative or a cultural occupation would be beneficial.

No deadlock on sleep
Really restful sleep is important for maintaining and maintaining a good memory.
Our brain takes advantage of the night, sleep to sort and organize the memories stored during the day.

MEMORY ENEMIES!
Insomnia, fatigue, depression, stress ... can disturb our memory. This is also the case of a traumatic event such as bereavement, loss of work or separation. Alcohol, caffeine, tobacco but also some drugs such as sleeping pills or anxiolytics are also disruptive.

Let's talk about stress
Cortisol is nicknamed the stress hormone because the body synthesizes it when it is in a state of stress. When its rate increases over a short period it has beneficial effects and makes more alert. But when one is exposed to long-term stress, high levels of cortisol also over a significant period can have negative effects, especially on what is called short-term memory.

1, 2, 3 let's go!
The brain acts like a muscle. Each physical or mental task stimulates the network of neurons and synaptic connections. This means that practicing physical activity and having multiple brain activities are ways to maintain your brain, train it, make it perform better and keep it in shape

SOME IDEAS
An energetic breakfast
• Take a large piece of wholemeal or sourdough bread with butter.
• Take piece of white or raw ham or an egg (fried, omelet or boiled).

- Take about 50g of hard cheese (Emmental cheese, cheese ...) or plain yoghurt.
- Eat a seasonal fruit.
- Drink Tea, coffee, herbal tea, water or fruit juice.

Give your brain the food it needs
To work well, the brain needs to be regularly supplied with fuel. In the morning, he has exhausted all his reserves ... We must renew them!
The midday meal should be rich in protein, meat or fish accompanied by green vegetables, starchy foods, a seasonal fruit.
The dinner should be light to promote a restful sleep.
As an accompaniment to a balanced diet, plant extracts such as Ginkgo biloba, Bacopa monnieri, DHA, a fatty acid from the omega 3 family can help maintain normal brain function and, in particular, memory.

In case of fasting, the brain can use medium chain triglycerides (MCTs) as an alternative fuel. In nature, medium chain triglycerides are abundantly present in coconut oil. They have interesting properties and are a rapidly available source of energy for the body, the brain, and the nervous system.
Vitamin B12 contributes to the proper functioning of the nervous system, normal energy metabolism, and normal psychological functions.

CHAPTER TEN

HOW YOUR COFFEE CAN MAKE YOUR BELLY BIG

Perkins researchers in Australia have shown that drinking too much coffee could make the metabolic syndrome worse
No, coffee does not make you lose weight. An Australian study published in the Journal of Agricultural and Food Chemistry shows that a compound present in coffee, known as chlorogenic acid (CGA) could worsen abdominal fatness.

How did they discover the abnormal retention of fat in the cells?
The scientists conducted their experiment on male mice for 12 weeks. They divided the rodents into four distinct groups: a group on a diet, the second group on a normal diet, a third on a high-fat diet, and the last group on a diet high in fat and acid. chlorogenic. The researchers wanted to evaluate the effect of CGA on obesity, glucose intolerance, insulin resistance, fatty acid oxidation and insulin signaling in male mice. The results showed that CGA would affect fat utilization in the liver and cause abnormal fat retention in belly cells. This study, therefore, suggests that supplementation with CGA in a high-fat diet does not protect against the characteristics of the metabolic syndrome. This syndrome refers to the presence of a set of physiological signs that increase the risk of type 2 diabetes, heart disease, and stroke. These physiological signs are abdominal overweight, high blood glucose, high triglyceride levels, high blood pressure and high cholesterol.

Advice: Do not exceed 3 to 4 cups of coffee a day
However, previous studies have shown that chlorogenic acid (CGA) has health benefits such as reduced body fat accumulation, reduced blood pressure, and increased insulin sensitivity but only at a certain dose. CGA is also one of the most consumed polyphenols in the diet because it is also found in some fruits such as plum. "The consumption of coffee reduces the risk of developing type 2 diabetes," said the study's lead author, Professor Kevin Croft, before continuing "With this in mind, we have studied the effects of polyphenols, or more especially CGAs previously known for their health benefits. " But researchers have discovered that beyond three or four cups of coffee, the beneficial effects on the body and on health have reversed.

Beware of coffee-based slimming products
Kevin Croft said: "A moderate intake of coffee, up to three to four cups a day, still seems to reduce the risk of developing diseases such as cardiovascular disease and type 2 diabetes, but it is important to remember that compounds such as CGA can have an effect on our health if they are not consumed in moderation ". The researcher also said that you should be wary of coffee-based slimming products: "People could lose their money if they buy expensive products such as dietary supplements of green coffee beans that are currently considered as products of incredible weight loss ".

CHAPTER ELEVEN

5 FOODS THAT PUMP OUR ENERGY
___

There are anti-fatigue foods ... and others, to avoid in case of total fatigue. We detail these enemies of well-being incoming lines.
The immune system, tension at half-mast, repetition of small nights: you are in small form, and you are looking for ways to re-boost your energy meter. These foods are to be avoided for a while if you do not want to exhaust your body.

In case of total fatigue, choose your oil
Temporarily eliminate oils rich in saturated fatty acids (the bad fat, such as rapeseed oil, palm oil or sunflower oil, which raise cholesterol levels in the blood and increase digestion) . Prefer unrefined oils, such as olive oil, rich in unsaturated fatty acids thathave positive effects on the cardiovascular system.

Intense fatigue? Avoid sweets drinks
The lack of sleep puts the bazaar in the secretion of the regulating hormones of the appetite. Since the body is lacking in energy, it secretes ghrelin, which stimulates the appetite, then leptin when it feels satiated.
These cravings often push us towards comforting foods, preferably sweet or fatty, which bring an interesting boost, then leave us even more emptied once the peak of insulin passed.
Sweets, cakes and other delicacies, rich in sugars, require a lot of energy to digest, which further depletes the already weak immune system. If the craving is too much for you, opt for fresh, vitamin-rich fruits or low-fat, unrefined sugar.

Avoid red meat
If proteins are necessary for our metabolism, it is better to favor other sources than red meat when we feel tired. In addition to being difficult to chew, digestion requires a lot of energy to the body when it does not have much.
Turn instead to lean meats (chicken, white meat) or fish, less rich and therefore less complex to digest.

The coffee, fake friend
When one is tired, the temptation is great to take the coffees to enjoy its whiplash effect. Except then, the peaks of glucose caused by its consumption leave the body even more weakened, and can cause the appearance of chronic fatigue. How to quench your thirst for energy? Drink tea instead! They stimulates the body, and you benefit from the long-term effects of the antioxidants it contains. Great

Put down your glass.
The digestion of alcohol, rich in sugars, requires a great effort on the part of the liver, which uses

a lot of energy to perform its cleaning work. Rather than adding extra hours to the liver by going down many glasses, it is better to avoid the alcohol the time to be re-boosted and to privilege the water, essential to eliminate the waste which clutches the cells.

CHAPTER TWELVE

TIPS TO EDUCATE YOUR CHILD TO FOLLOW THE RULES.

In life, we cannot do everything. There are rules to follow. Here are some tips on how to educate your child and teach him/her to follow the instructions, and obey in first place parental authority or another one.

Educate your child: Not easy to pass parental authority.
It is that the stake is of size. It is neither more nor less to make a little being who will both respect the rules of life in society and flourish.
"We do not civilize a child, we give him frames to help him civilize himself, says psychoanalyst Claude Halmos. Learning the laws of the world is not only with the head but also with the body, the heart, the emotions.

Just as concrete is made of cement, the child is built with the law. She becomes an integral part of him. And note: "We can have children who have learned the rules from the outside without having integrated them internally. In adolescence, these children who were said to be so well educated transgress the law. "
Hence the importance of appealing to your child's understanding rather than imposing rules that make no sense to him. To obtain his adhesion rather than pour it into a mold. To teach him to obey rather than to submit.
Still, the exercise of authority is rarely a part of pleasure. Refusing his child what he wants, impose prohibitions on him, it is always a little pain. And no father/mother likes that.
"In life, everything is not possible and it's frustrating," says the psychoanalyst. But it's also liberating. The child who is put on limits will stop living in the illusion that he can always have more, and thus stop feeling unhappy and unloved. Because a child who thinks he can always get more believes that if we do not give him what he wants, it's because we do not like him. "

Educate your child: from 2 years, tell him that there is a limit. We cannot do everything.
To be able to live in society, your child must integrate three fundamental prohibitions:
1. You cannot be the husband/wife of your father/mother . Therefore, you do not go to bed with your parents and let them kiss without anger or try to separate them. If you let go, you validate the incest fantasy of your child , who knows no limit then ...
2. Do not hit the other. Explain it simply: "Your dad does not hit the neighbor every time he increases his TV volume or lets his trash bag hang out in front of the door. You do not slap on your boyfriend because he pissed you off. "
3. We do not have what the other has. We do not seize his toys, we do not spoil his clothes, etc. because it belongs to him and it would hurt him. It's all about getting the message across do not do to others what you do not want us to do to you.

The problem is that, to be able to represent what the other feels, it is necessary that your child has acquired a certain independence on the motor level. That he knows how to manage without the help of anyone in all the little things of everyday life: getting up, going to the bathroom, eating, etc. "Integrate the law, it works with autonomy. You cannot ask a child to do it before 2-3 years," says Claude Halmos.

Educate your child: It is easier to educate with examples. Give him examples.
Explain to your child that you too, have obligations. You cannot walk naked on the street, or buy anything that tempts you. Your child will accept more of the limitations you give him when he understands that you too are accountable.
"A child is built by taking his parents as models," recalls Claude -Halmos. The least of your gestures is a message. If only for road safety, parents are often blamed: they often set a bad example for their children.

Educate your child: make sure the prohibitions are respected.
Even if you have prohibited, it is difficult for your child to give up the satisfaction of his wishes. He also needs to test the barriers you have put in place.
It's up to you to show him that you are ready to enforce them! "A child is very aware of the determination and conviction of the adult," observes Claude Halmos.
Explain to him the reason for your request once (you do not tear off this toy from your brother's hands, it's up to him to decide if he will lend it to you), possibly twice if he does not seem have understood correctly.
But, in the third, be firm: "You heard me very well, now you do what I ask you, that's all. He does not obey? You have the right to show your anger. Announce what will happen: "You know the rule, you will be punished. "
Above all, do not go into endless explanations, you do not have to win at all costs. The more you discuss, the more he will seek to negotiate.

Educate your child: what punishment to choose if he does not obey?
"It's up to each parent to decide, according to their child," says psychoanalyst Claude Halmos. It must of course that the penalty annoys him, otherwise it has no value. It must also be adapted to the fault, neither too severe nor not enough. "
It may just be "now you're going to your room" if you feel like that. "The punishment that will work is that the parent feels able to hold, the one he assumes feeling legitimate," continues Claude Halmos.
If the parent feels that he is hurting his child, it will not work. He will be uncomfortable, he will not have the necessary conviction and the child will feel that there is a possible escape. "

Educate your child: and if he still does not respect the rules?
You have set the rules but nothing to do! Your little one does not respect them. "A child who transgresses systematically can be a child who has difficulties that he cannot say otherwise," observes Claude Halmos.
If your little one constantly disobeys and does stupid things, take the time to talk with him. Listening to him will enable him to become aware of his behavior and to gradually express his anxieties by words instead of putting them into action. "

But, more often than not, a child who constantly disobeys is a child who feels cracks in the barriers that his parents have erected , says the psychoanalyst.
This is usually related to what the parent himself has experienced. Either he did not receive limits when he was small, and he has trouble finding the marks to give to his child. On the contrary, he has the memory of being a victim of the tyranny of adults, subjected to arbitrary, humiliated, and, consciously or unconsciously, he is afraid to impose the same thing on his child. "
Whatever the problem, do not hesitate to consult a therapist. A few sessions may be enough to resolve the situation.

Educate your child: 9 mistakes not to do.
1 - Believe your child will understand and learn the rules alone. He needs you to educate him to grow.
2 - Think that because you explained the rules, it is no longer necessary to impose them. A fighting phase is inevitable.
3 - All forbid. The "all-forbidden" is not only destructive but also counterproductive.
4 - Give orders without explaining, train your child to obey.
5 - Promise a punishment and not give it. You lose all credibility. Next time, he'll look at you with a smirk.
6 - Forbid one day, allow the next day. Your child needs consistency, otherwise, he does not understand anything.
7 - Be terrorized at the thought of hurting your little one. Of course, you impose frustrations on him. But these are normal and inevitable sufferings. It's the same when you ask him not to put his hand in the socket!
8 - Imagine that because you forbid something to your child, you are a bad parent. To love is to educate, on the contrary. ,
9 - To assimilate your child to his actions. . He stole a trinket at the supermarket? There is no point in humiliating him by calling him a thief. We must explain to him what theft is, tell him that he is punished by society and warn him that he himself will be punished if he starts again.

CHAPTER THIRTEEN

BE CAREFUL: CARBONATED WATER CAN MAKE YOU HUNGRY.

JPsante hopes that you have entered very well into 2018. You have started working in order to make your 2018 year resolution a reality at the end of 2018. I guess one of them is to have a healthy life.
JPsante will be by your side by providing you the necessary health information you need.
Now it is like almost our foods especially industrial foods and drinks are likely to make us obese. It is a must for everyone that in one way, eats or drinks them on the regular basis to be careful.

On that note, *British researchers warn against drinks containing bubbles, including sparkling water, which would increase hunger by 50% and push to eat more.*
Gizzard, liver, turkey, chestnuts, ... You have enjoyed the holiday meals of the end of years and like many other people now you intend to pay attention to your food after the excesses? Be careful not to overuse the sparkling water used very often in case of diet because it helps those who are addicted to sodas to hold the blow in case of diet. According to the BBC2 column "Trust me I am a doctor", relayed by the Dailymail, gas bubbles in the sparkling water would promote hunger.

How have they arrived at the 50% of risk of hunger?
Scientists had established at the time that it is not only because of sugar that sodas make you fat but also because of bubbles. Suddenly, the authors (University of Birzeit (United Kingdom)) of the Chronicle decided to know if it was the case for the gas water. "We asked several volunteers to fast for 10 hours and then put the same amount of calories in. An hour later some had to drink a soda, some gas water and some of the water, "says Dr. Michael Mosley in the *Dailymail*.

Scientists then conducted blood tests on volunteers to assess their levels of ghrelin, also known as the 'hunger hormone', which transmits information from the stomach to the brain when it comes to eating. Those who drank a drink with bubbles, the rate of ghrelin was raised by 50% compared to those who drank water ", reports the author. They would have also consumed 120 calories more.

Takeaways
Researchers do not yet know why bubbles would have such an effect on hunger. They propose two hypotheses: either the bubbles of gas in the drink would have directly a ghrelin trigger, or the stomach swells in contact with the gas bubbles and gets bigger which causes the diffusion of the hormone of the hunger towards the brain. Even if the results are minimal the specialists recommend to those who consume a lot to reduce the intake of beverage containing bubbles.

CHAPTER FORTEEN

WHAT IS PRECONCEPTION CONSULTATION AND WHY IS IT SO IMPORTANT STEP?

Many pregnancy complications can be avoided if the couples have given to preconception consultation an important step. Consult before conceiving a baby may be useful in some cases to ensure that the expected pregnancy is not going to be a problem. Who is this consultation for? Who to consult? Let us find out.

The desire for a child is a personal, intimate wish that belongs to the couple. The project of pregnancy, its hope of realization, are part of the natural events of their life and to consult a doctor on this subject does not appear to them necessary. Pre-conception consultation may, however, be useful for some women who wish to become pregnant; it will be an opportunity to ensure that the expected pregnancy will not be a problem for their health and that of their future baby.

In which medical situations is it reasonable to ask for an opinion and to whom?

• If you have an illness that requires continued treatment, tell your doctor about your desire for a child. If he does not tell you about it, it's not because he thinks that a pregnancy would be bad for you, it's probably because he does not anticipate this project for you. He will then direct you to the most suitable professional.

• The gynecologist-obstetrician is best placed to give an opinion. You can also consult it without mail from your doctor. In certain special cases, the gynecologist-obstetrician will take the advice of fellow specialists, such as a cardiologist, a diabetologist, a neurologist, a psychiatrist, especially if you are hypertensive, diabetic, or treated for epilepsy or for psychiatric disorders.

• If you have any of these conditions, you are probably aware of the potential risks of pregnancy, and it is particularly important to monitor or modify the current treatment; it is the same in case of heart disease. But do not modify or interrupt your treatment without medical advice: this is what some women do, fearing that their treatment will be harmful to their baby if a pregnancy occurs. Thus, in case of diabetes, it is important that glycemic be as balanced as possible several months before fertilization. This reduces the risk of complications.

What To know about the preconception consultation?

• There are other medical situations in which it is highly recommended to have medical advice, which women do not always know. This is the case of obesity, asthma, a history of thrombosis, diseases of the thyroid gland or autoimmune diseases such as lupus.

• If you have ever been pregnant and have had complications such as recurrent miscarriage, the loss of a baby during pregnancy or at the time of birth, premature delivery, if you had a particular cesarean section because of preeclampsia: again it is advisable to consult an obstetrician; it is the same if you know that you have a uterine malformation, or if your mother has taken distilbene.

• Preconception consultation is advised, apart from any pathology, if you are 40 years old or older. The doctor will perform a general examination, including cardiology, more complete.

• Also, be aware that there are genetics consultations in major hospitals and that every time a genetic risk is known in the family, you will be told the level of risk of having the same disease and if it can be detected before birth.

CHAPTER FIFTEEN

DO NOT GIVE CODEINE OR TRAMADOL TO A CHILD

According to the US FDA, these two drugs can put the lives of some children at risk.
Codeine and tramadol should not be used to treat pain or a cough in children under 12 years of age as they can lead to fatal accidents, the US Food and Drug Administration (FDA) announced on 20 April.
The FDA has unveiled several changes in the drug product leaflets that use these substances to protect children, teens, and breastfed infants.

"Some children who have received codeine or tramadol have experienced a fatal respiratory distress syndrome because they metabolize synthetic drugs much more quickly, which leads to dangerously high levels of the active ingredient in their body," says the FDA in a statement.

FDA ADDS NEW RESTRICTIONS:
- Codeine is contraindicated for treating pain or a cough and tramadol is contraindicated for the treatment of pain in children under 12 years of age
- Tramadol is contraindicated for the treatment of pain after removal of tonsils.
- Codeine and tramadol are not recommended for adolescents aged 12 to 18 who are obese or have conditions such as sleep apnea or severe lung disease.
- Mothers should not breast-feed while taking codeine or tramadol.

Since 1969, codeine has been linked in the US to 64 cases of serious respiratory problems, including 24 deaths in children and adolescents. Tramadol has been linked to 9 cases of severe respiratory problems, including 3 deaths in children and adolescents. There were cases of respiratory problems in breastfed infants whose mothers were taking codeine

CHAPTER SIXTEEN

HOW TO CHANGE THE AGE OF YOUR HEART

Livescience presents new results from an American study that demonstrates a link between reducing heart failure and increasing physical activity.

if a simple way could allow you to rejuvenate your heart? According to a study presented in the United States on November 11, there is one: to play sports. According to Dr. Roberta Florido, co-author of the research at Johns Hopkins University School in Baltimore : "Physical activity could prevent the development of the" little thick heart "associated with heart failure."

Beneficial changes in the cardiac structure
In their analysis of 9427 participants, scientists assessed the association between physical activity and chronic myocardial injury. They then selected 2700 people who performed an MRI of their heart at the beginning of the study and 10 years later. The participants averaged about 60 years at the start of the study, all of whom gave accurate information about their physical activity levels.

Results : During the 10 years of study, an increase in physical activity was significantly related to beneficial changes in the participants' cardiac structure. They observed an increase in cardiac volume and a maintenance of the thickness of the cardiac wall when the participants were doing sports.

75 minutes of activity per week
On *Livescience* , Dr. Roberta Florido explains, "Often, as people get older, the walls of their heart become thicker, while their heart cavities become smaller. This" small thick heart "increases the risk of heart failure. , a condition in which the heart muscle cannot pump enough blood to meet the body's normal demands. " The thick walls of the heart prevent the normal function of the pump and increase the risk of developing heart failure. To maintain the thickness of the walls and keep a heart in shape, the best solution would be to increase physical activity. "I recommend people to practice 150 minutes of moderate activity, or 75 minutes of vigorous activity, per week," Dr. Florido advised.

CHAPTER SEVENTEEN

WHAT ARE THE VITAMINS AND MINERALS FOR CHILDREN BETWEEN 1 TO 3 YEARS OLD?

Several vitamins and minerals are essential for the growth and development of your child. The best way to ensure that these nutritional needs are met is to provide a varied and balanced diet. The dark green vegetables, as well as the fruits and vegetables oranged, are to be included most often on the menu, that is to say, every day! In addition, vegetables and fresh fruits are encouraged and, if possible, with their peel.
Here are some of the essential nutrients and their roles:
• Vitamins (vitamin A, vitamin C, vitamin D)
• Minerals (calcium, iron, magnesium, phosphorus, zinc)

Let's start with VITAMINS

VITAMIN A
WHERE TO GET VITAMIN A?
Liver (chicken, beef, etc.)and fish liver oil, Leafy green vegetables, Orange fruits, and vegetables,
including cantaloupe, mango, and sweet potato, Eggs, Dairy products

WHY VITAMIN A?
JPsante: Vitamin A allows the growth of bones and tissues covering various parts of the body (cornea, bronchi, intestine, skin ...). It allows to see well at night and contributes to the proper functioning of the immune system.

VITAMIN C
WHERE TO GET VITAMIN C?
Green, yellow and red peppers, Strawberries, raspberries, kiwis, melons, mangoes, Oranges, grapefruit, clementines, mandarins
Tomatoes, turnips, potatoes with peel, spinach, Cauliflower, broccoli, Brussels sprout, Juices of fruits and vegetables

WHY VITAMIN C?
JPsante: Vitamin C increases iron absorption from grain products, legumes, eggs, and vegetables. It helps the immune system function, heal wounds and maintain skin integrity.
Vitamin C is very sensitive: light, heat, and air can destroy it. To preserve it, you must not cook vegetables too much and cut fruits too far in advance.

VITAMIN D
WHERE TO GET VITAMIN D?
Milk, enriched yogurt, Fortified soy beverages, Fat fish and fish oils

WHERE TO GET VITAMIN D?
JPsante: Vitamin D contributes to the health of bones and teeth by facilitating the absorption of calcium and normalizing blood calcium and phosphorus levels. It also contributes to several functions in the body such as strengthening the immune system. Studies have also concluded that it will help prevent certain cancers.

Thanks to the sun, the body creates its own vitamin D. About ten minutes of skin exposure in the midday sun (without sunscreen) would be enough to meet the needs of children. The problem is that in some parts of the world, the sun and the power of the sun are insufficient from October to April.

However, it is difficult to achieve the recommended intake of vitamin D by diet alone. That's why more and more pediatricians and nutritionists recommend that children take a supplement of 400 IU during the fall and winter, in addition to their two daily glasses of milk. Breastfed babies should also be supplemented with 400 IU of vitamin D a day, breast milk does not contain enough.

MINERALS

CALCIUM
WHERE TO GET CALCIUM?
Dairy products (milk, yogurt, cheese ...), Fortified soy beverages, Almonds, Fish (salmon, sardine) canned with bones
Green vegetables (broccoli, cabbage ...)

WHY CALCIUM?
JPsante: Calcium helps build and maintain strong bones and teeth. It is also essential for muscle contractions, including those of the heart. It helps regulate blood pressure and promotes healing.

IRON
WHERE TO GET IRON?
Meat, Poultry, Seafood, eggs, legumes, Cereal products fortified with iron, Dark green vegetables, Nuts and seeds

WHY IRON?
JPsante: Iron exists in two forms: hemic and non-heme. Heme iron in meat, poultry, and fish is better absorbed than non-heme iron provided by eggs and vegetables. When there is no meat or fish in the meal, you can include a vitamin C-containing food that increases the absorption of non-heme iron.

Iron transports oxygen to the cells of tissues and muscles. It also facilitates the cognitive development of young people by increasing their attention and concentration and improving their intellectual performance.

MAGNESIUM
WHERE TO GET MAGNESIUM?
Green vegetables, legumes, Nuts and seeds, Whole grain cereal products

WHY MAGNESIUM?
JPsante: Magnesium helps the solidification of bones and teeth. It also helps the muscles and the heart to do their job well and participates in more than 300 functions in the body.

PHOSPHORUS
WHERE TO GET PHOSPHORUS?
Meat, eggs, Fish, Dairy products, Nuts and seeds, Legumes (lentils, beans, and peas)

WHY PHOSPHORUS?
JPsante: Phosphorus plays a role in the formation of bones and teeth. It also helps to produce and store the energy the body needs, and a host of other chemical reactions inside every cell.

ZINC
WHERE TO GET ZINC?
Red meats, poultry, legumes, Nuts, seafood, Whole grain cereal products, Dairy products

WHY ZINC?
JPsante: Zinc from meat, poultry and seafood is better absorbed than from cereals, legumes or vegetables.it allows the development and growth of toddlers. It helps fight infections and wound healing.

BEWARE OF SUFFOCATION!
As the diameter of the esophagus of young children is small, they are more likely to be choked. Peanuts, crunchy peanut butter, nuts and unmilled seeds are therefore to be avoided. Give your child nuts and ground seeds until he is 4 years old.

Foods provide several other essential vitamins and minerals such as potassium, selenium, folate, vitamin B12, and so on. These nutrients are found in various foods. There is no complete food or that guarantees health on its own. That's why the best way to make sure your kids do not miss anything is to offer them a varied diet.

www.ingramcontent.com/pod-product-compliance
Lightning Source LLC
Chambersburg PA
CBHW030601220526
45463CB00007B/3136